101

HERBAL REMEDIES YOU SHOULD KNOW

Inspired by Barbara O'Neill's Teachings.

Niella Brown

Disclaimer:

The information provided in this book is for informational purposes only. Please consult with your health care provider for medical advice. The author specifically disclaims any liability that is incurred from the use or application of the contents of this book

Inspired By Barbara Oneill's Teachings

Get Exclusive Access To all Barbara O'Neill's Videos, Lectures and Teachings.

Scan the Code Below to get Started.

Table of Contents

INTRODUCTION

EMBRACING NATURE'S PHARMACY: A JOURNEY INTO HERBAL HEALING

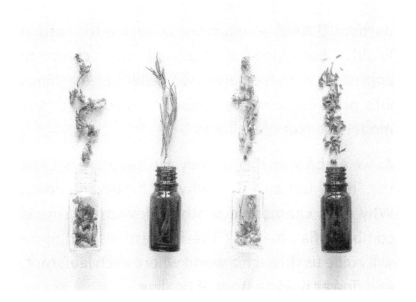

Welcome to "101 Herbal Remedies You Should Know Before 2025," a guide that bridges the time-honored wisdom of herbal healing with contemporary understanding. This book is not just a collection of herbal formulas; it is an invitation to explore the profound relationship between nature and our health, inspired by the holistic teachings of Barbara O'Neill.

In an age where quick fixes and synthetic solutions often take precedence, we turn our gaze back to the gentle yet powerful world of herbs. Here, healing is more than just addressing symptoms; it's about nurturing a deep connection with our bodies and the natural world.

Barbara O'Neill, a renowned advocate for natural health, has long championed this complete approach. In these pages, we distill her teachings into practical, accessible wisdom, tailored for the modern seeker of wellness.

As we embark on this journey, we'll explore not just the "how" but also the "why" of herbal remedies. Why does chamomile soothe? How can turmeric combat inflammation? These questions and more will guide us through a world where each leaf, root, and flower holds a story of healing.

But this book is more than a mere guide. It's a call to embrace a whole lifestyle, where our choices - from the food we eat to the remedies we use - are in harmony with nature. It's about understanding that true wellness is a fabric woven from the threads of physical health, mental clarity, emotional balance, and spiritual well-being.

Whether you are new to herbal remedies or an experienced practitioner, this book is designed to enrich your understanding and inspire a deeper engagement with your health. Each page is infused with the wisdom of traditional practices and scientific research, ensuring that you have the most reliable and up-to-date information at your fingertips.

As you turn these pages, remember that each remedy is more than a prescription; it's a conversation with nature. A dialogue between the ancient wisdom of our ancestors and the needs of our modern lives. So, let us begin this journey with open hearts and curious minds, as we unlock the secrets of nature's pharmacy and weave a new narrative of health and healing for ourselves and our world.

Welcome to the journey. Welcome to "101 Herbal Remedies You Should Know Before 2025."

CHAPTER 1: FOUNDATIONS OF HERBAL HEALING

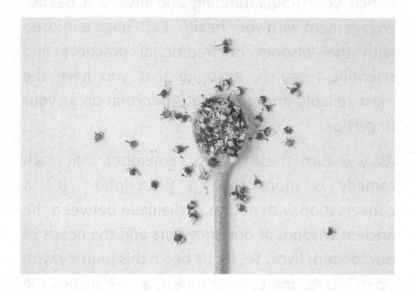

Foundations of Herbal Healing form the cornerstone of understanding and effectively using herbal remedies. This concept is rooted in the ancient tradition of using plants for medicinal purposes, a practice that has evolved over centuries across various cultures. It's not just about the herbs themselves, but about a whole approach to health, emphasizing the balance and harmony of the body, mind, and environment.

At its core, the foundation of herbal healing is built upon the principle that nature offers the necessary tools to heal and maintain a healthy body. Each herb possesses unique properties and active ingredients that interact with the body's systems, facilitating healing and promoting wellness. The efficacy of these remedies is often attributed to the synergy of their components, which work together to enhance their therapeutic effects.

Understanding herbal healing also involves a deep appreciation of the body's natural healing processes. It's about recognizing the body's innate ability to heal itself and how herbs can support and accelerate this process. This perspective requires a shift from merely treating symptoms to addressing the underlying causes of ailments, fostering a more holistic approach to health.

Another key aspect is the knowledge of herb identification, harvesting, and preparation. Knowing how to identify the right herbs, understanding their life cycles, and learning the appropriate times for harvesting to ensure potency is crucial. Equally important is mastering the various methods of preparation, such as creating tinctures, teas, and salves, which can vary significantly depending on the intended use of the herb.

Safety and understanding potential interactions with other medications and conditions are also fundamental. This includes being aware of any contraindications, understanding the appropriate dosages, and recognizing the limits of herbal remedies. While these remedies are natural, they are not without risks, and educating oneself about these aspects is essential for safe and effective use.

Lastly, the foundations of herbal healing are deeply connected to a broader holistic lifestyle. This involves a commitment to overall wellness, including a balanced diet, regular exercise, and stress management. Herbs are seen not just as remedies for specific ailments but as part of a larger strategy for maintaining health and preventing disease.

In essence, the foundations of herbal healing are a blend of ancient wisdom and modern understanding, emphasizing a respectful and informed relationship with the natural world. It's about seeing herbs not just as tools for treatment, but as allies in a lifelong journey toward health and well-being

The Basics of Herbal Medicine

Herbal medicine, at its core, is the use of plants to promote health and treat illness. This practice dates back thousands of years and forms a crucial part of traditional medicine systems worldwide. In herbalism, each plant is believed to possess unique properties and can be used to treat specific health conditions.

Herbs can be used in various forms: as raw ingredients, teas, tinctures, extracts, oils, or salves. The choice of form depends on the herb and the condition being treated. For example, chamomile might be used as a tea for relaxation, while echinacea could be taken as a tincture to boost immunity.

One of the fundamental principles of herbal medicine is the concept of synergy. This principle suggests that the therapeutic effect of the whole herb, with all its components, is greater than its isolated active ingredients. This integrated approach contrasts with conventional medicine, which often focuses on single, isolated compounds.

History and Evolution of Herbal Remedies

Herbal remedies have evolved through centuries, intertwined with the history and culture of various civilizations. Ancient texts from China, India, Egypt, and Greece all document the extensive use of herbal remedies. The Ebers Papyrus from ancient Egypt, for example, lists over 850 herbal prescriptions.

Over time, the knowledge of herbal remedies spread across continents. The Middle Ages saw herbalism flourish in Europe, with monasteries playing a crucial role in preserving this knowledge. The Renaissance further advanced herbal medicine, with botanists like Nicholas Culpeper publishing detailed herbals.

The Industrial Revolution and the rise of synthetic pharmaceuticals saw a decline in the use of herbal remedies in the West. However, there has been a resurgence in interest in recent decades, driven by a desire for natural and complete approaches to health.

Understanding Your Body and Its Needs

Herbal medicine is deeply rooted in the understanding that each person's body has unique needs and responses. This perspective emphasizes the importance of individualized treatment. Factors such as age, lifestyle, diet, and overall health play a crucial role in determining the most effective herbal remedies for an individual.

In this approach, the body is seen not just as a collection of symptoms to be treated but as a complex system that requires balance and harmony. For instance, an herbalist might recommend ginger not just for its ability to alleviate nausea but also for its warming properties that can balance a 'cold' condition in the body.

The Principles of Holistic Wellness

Holistic wellness is a comprehensive approach to health, considering the physical, emotional, mental, and spiritual aspects of an individual. It's about maintaining balance and harmony within oneself and with the surrounding environment.

In holistic wellness, prevention is key. It involves adopting a lifestyle that supports health, such as eating nutritious foods, getting regular exercise, managing stress, and fostering positive relationships.

Herbal remedies play a significant role in holistic wellness. They are not just used for treating illness but also for maintaining health and preventing disease. For instance, adaptogenic herbs like ashwagandha are used to help the body resist stressors of all kinds, whether physical, chemical, or biological.

By embracing these principles, herbal medicine offers a natural, gentle, and effective way to support health and well-being, in line with the philosophies of experts like Barbara O'Neill. This approach encourages individuals to take an active role in their health, using the healing powers of nature as a guide and a tool for wellness.

CHAPTER 2: PREPARING HERBAL REMEDIES

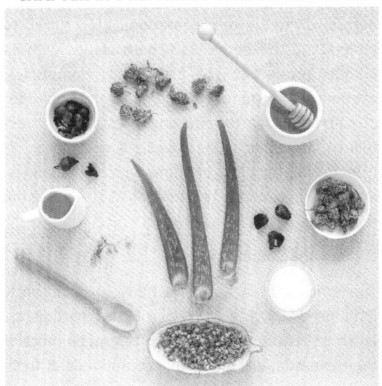

Preparing herbal remedies is an art that intertwines with science, a practice deeply rooted in our history and yet ever-evolving. The art of crafting these remedies requires not only knowledge of the herbs themselves but also an understanding of their synergy with the human body and mind. This journey into the world of herbal remedies illuminates a path towards natural health and holistic wellness.

Understanding the Herbs

Before diving into preparation, it's crucial to understand the herbs. Each herb comes with its unique properties, benefits, and, sometimes, cautions. For instance, chamomile is renowned for its calming properties, making it a staple in stress relief remedies. Meanwhile, echinacea is celebrated for its immune-boosting abilities. Knowing these characteristics helps in selecting the right herb for the right ailment.

Quality and Sourcing

The efficacy of a herbal remedy is significantly influenced by the quality of its ingredients. Freshness is key - fresh herbs often retain more of their essential oils and active compounds. If fresh herbs aren't accessible, dried herbs are a viable alternative, provided they are well-preserved and of good quality.

Sourcing herbs responsibly is also vital. Ethical and sustainable sourcing ensures the longevity of plant species and respects the environment. Moreover, organically grown herbs, free from pesticides and chemicals, contribute to a healthier product.

Preparing Herbal Remedies

The process of preparing herbal remedies varies based on the desired outcome and the specific characteristics of the herbs used. Here are some common methods:

1. **Infusions and Teas:** Perhaps the simplest form of herbal remedy, infusions involve steeping herbs in hot water. This method is most suitable for delicate parts of the plant, like leaves and flowers. Green tea, known for its antioxidant properties, is a classic example.

2. **Decoctions:** For tougher plant parts like roots, bark, and seeds, decoctions are more appropriate. This involves simmering the herb in water over a longer period, allowing the extraction of its potent compounds. Ginger tea, made from the root, is an excellent decoy for digestion and inflammation.

3. **Tinctures:** Tinctures are concentrated herbal extracts made by soaking herbs in alcohol or vinegar. This method extracts the active compounds effectively and extends the shelf life of the remedy. Echinacea tincture is a popular choice for immune support.

4. **Ointments and Salves:** For topical applications, herbs can be infused into oils or mixed with waxes to create ointments and salves. These are particularly useful for skin conditions, wounds, or muscle aches. Calendula salve is a go-to for skin irritations and minor cuts.

5. **Capsules and Powders:** Some prefer their herbs in capsules or powders for ease of consumption and precise dosage. This method often requires dried and ground herbs. Turmeric, with its anti-inflammatory properties, is frequently consumed in capsule form.

Dosage and Safety

While natural, herbal remedies are not without their risks. Proper dosages should be respected, as even natural substances can be harmful in excessive amounts. Additionally, it's important to consider potential allergies and interactions with other medications. Consulting with a healthcare provider, especially for those with existing health conditions, is always recommended.

The Holistic Approach

Herbal remedies are not just about treating symptoms; they are part of a broader, holistic approach to health. This philosophy emphasizes the balance of mind, body, and spirit. Incorporating herbal remedies into a lifestyle that values a balanced diet, regular exercise, and stress management amplifies their effectiveness.

The Role of Mindfulness and Intention

The process of preparing herbal remedies can be a meditative and mindful practice. Engaging with the herbs, understanding their origins, and preparing them with intention can create a deeper connection to the natural world and our wellness journey.

Continuing Education and Experimentation

The field of herbal medicine is vast and ever-expanding. Continual learning and experimentation are key to mastering the art of herbal remedy preparation. Attending workshops, reading extensively, and joining communities can enhance one's knowledge and skills.

In conclusion, preparing herbal remedies is a journey that offers more than just physical health benefits; it is a gateway to a more connected and harmonious way of living. It's a practice that calls for respect for nature, a commitment to learning, and a mindfulness that transcends the act of preparation itself. Embracing this ancient yet evolving art can lead to a fulfilling path in natural health and holistic wellness.

Selecting Quality Herbs

Selecting quality herbs is a fundamental step in embracing natural health principles and holistic practices for self-healing and wellness. The potency, purity, and efficacy of herbal remedies largely depend on the quality of the herbs used. In this comprehensive guide, we'll delve into various aspects of selecting quality herbs, and blending traditional wisdom with modern insights to ensure you make informed choices in your journey toward natural health.

Understanding Herb Quality

1. Source and Origin: The origin of herbs plays a crucial role in their quality. Herbs grown in their native environment tend to have a higher potency. For example, ginseng from East Asia and Echinacea from North America are known for their superior quality due to the optimal growing conditions in these regions.

2. Organic vs. Non-Organic: Organic herbs are grown without synthetic pesticides, herbicides, and fertilizers. These herbs are often preferred for their purity and minimal exposure to harmful chemicals. Organic certification, although not always feasible for all herbs, is a reliable indicator of quality.

3. Wildcrafted Herbs: Wildcrafting involves gathering herbs from their natural, wild habitat. These herbs are valued for their robustness and high active ingredient content. However, ethical and sustainable harvesting practices are essential to protect these natural resources.

Evaluating Physical Characteristics

4. Appearance: Healthy, quality herbs have a vibrant color indicative of their freshness and potency. Faded, discolored, or moldy herbs are signs of poor quality.

5. Aroma and Flavor: A strong, distinct aroma is a hallmark of a quality herb. Similarly, the flavor should be pronounced – bitterness in dandelion roots or the pungency of ginger indicates freshness and potency.

6. Texture: Properly dried herbs should have a crisp texture. If they feel overly dry and crumbly or, conversely, too moist, it may signal improper handling and storage.

Understanding Harvesting and Processing

7. Harvesting Time: The time of harvest is pivotal. Many herbs have specific harvesting periods when their active constituents are at their peak. For instance, calendula flowers are best harvested in full bloom, while roots like valerian are often harvested in the fall.

8. Drying and Processing: The drying process should retain the herb's essential properties. Overheating or prolonged exposure to sunlight during drying can degrade the herb's active compounds. Proper drying techniques preserve both the physical and medicinal qualities of the herb.

9. Storage and Shelf Life: Quality herbs are stored in a way that preserves their potency. This typically means cool, dark, and dry conditions. Exposure to heat, light, and moisture can lead to deterioration. Be aware of the shelf life of herbs, as potency diminishes over time.

Ethical and Sustainable Practices

10. Sustainable Sourcing: Opt for herbs from sources that practice sustainable harvesting to ensure environmental conservation and the long-term availability of herbal resources.

11. Ethical Considerations: Be mindful of the ethical implications of herb sourcing. Some herbs are overharvested, leading to ecological imbalance or exploitation of local communities.

Navigating the Market

12. Reputable Suppliers: Purchasing herbs from reputable suppliers or growers is essential. Look for suppliers who provide detailed information about the herb's origin, processing, and storage.

13. Understanding Labels: Learn to decipher labels on herbal products. Terms like "standardized extract," "whole herb," and "certified organic" have specific meanings that can guide your selection.

14. Price as an Indicator: While price should not be the sole determinant of quality, exceptionally cheap herbs might indicate compromised quality. Investing in higher-quality herbs can lead to better health outcomes.

Personal Connection and Intuition

15. Intuition and Personal Connection: Sometimes, selecting herbs can also be an intuitive process. Trust your senses and intuition. The herbs that you feel drawn to might be the ones your body needs.

16. Experimentation and Learning: Herbalism is an ongoing learning experience. Experiment with different herbs and observe how your body responds to them. This personal experience is invaluable in understanding what works best for you.

Selecting quality herbs is an art and a science, requiring knowledge, mindfulness, and sometimes intuition. By understanding the factors that contribute to an herb's quality and embracing ethical and sustainable practices, we can ensure that the herbal remedies we use are not only effective but also in harmony with nature and our bodies. In the realm of natural health and holistic wellness, the quality of our herbs is not just a matter of efficacy; it's a reflection of our values and our commitment to nurturing ourselves and the world around us.

The preparation of herbal remedies is both an art and a science. Herbs, those humble plants that have been the cornerstone of traditional medicine for centuries, can be transformed into potent remedies through various methods. Each preparation technique, be it tinctures, teas, or other forms, has its unique benefits and applications. Understanding these methods not only empowers us to take control of our health naturally but also connects us deeply with the age-old practices of herbal healing.

1. The Art of Tinctures: Concentrated Herbal Power

Tinctures are one of the most effective and long-lasting ways to extract and preserve the medicinal properties of herbs. A tincture is essentially a concentrated herbal extract made by soaking herbs in alcohol or vinegar. The process, known as maceration, pulls out the active compounds from the plant material.

Why Tinctures?

- **Concentration**: Tinctures are highly concentrated, meaning you need only a small amount to achieve the desired effect.

- **Longevity**: The alcohol or vinegar preserves the extract, extending its shelf life significantly.

- **Rapid Absorption**: Being liquid, tinctures are quickly absorbed, offering faster relief than other forms.

Making Tinctures at Home

- Select high-quality, dried herbs.

- Chop or grind the herbs to increase the surface area.

- Place the herbs in a jar and cover them with alcohol (usually vodka or brandy for their neutral flavors) or apple cider vinegar.

- Seal the jar and store it in a cool, dark place, shaking it daily.

- After 4-6 weeks, strain the mixture and store the liquid in amber dropper bottles.

2. Herbal Teas: Simplicity and Tradition

Herbal teas, also known as infusions, are perhaps the simplest and most traditional method of herbal preparation. They involve steeping herbs in hot water to extract their medicinal properties.

Benefits of Herbal Teas

- **Ease of Preparation**: Making herbal tea is as simple as pouring hot water over herbs.

- **Hydration**: They provide a hydrating way to consume herbs.

- **Variety and Taste**: There's an endless variety of teas for every palate and condition.

Preparing Herbal Teas

- Boil water and pour it over the herb (loose or in a teabag) in a cup.

- Cover and steep for about 10-15 minutes.

- Strain (if using loose herbs) and enjoy. Sweeteners like honey can be added.

3. Herbal Powders: Versatility and Convenience

Herbal powders are made by finely grinding dried herbs. They are incredibly versatile and can be used in capsules, added to food, or mixed into drinks.

Advantages of Herbal Powders

- **Easy to Store and Transport**: Powders have a long shelf life and are easy to carry.

- **Versatility**: They can be incorporated into various recipes, making them an excellent option for those who dislike the taste of tinctures or teas.

Making and Using Herbal Powders

- Dry the herbs completely and grind them into a fine powder using a grinder.

- Store in airtight containers.

- Use them in capsules, or smoothies, or sprinkle them on food.

4. Herbal Oils and Salves: For External Healing

Herbal oils and salves are used topically for a range of skin conditions, aches, and pains. They involve infusing herbs in oils which are then used as is or turned into salves by adding beeswax.

Making Herbal Oils and Salves

- For oils, herbs are soaked in carrier oils like olive or coconut oil and left to infuse.

- For salves, the infused oil is gently heated with beeswax until it melts, then poured into containers to solidify.

5. Syrups and Elixirs: Sweet Herbal Preparations

Syrups and elixirs are sweetened herbal preparations, often used for their soothing effect on the throat and cough relief.

Preparing Syrups and Elixirs

- Make a strong herbal tea or decoction.

- Add honey or sugar, and simmer until it forms a syrupy consistency.

- Elixirs may also contain alcohol for preservation.

6. Herbal Baths: Soothing and Therapeutic

Herbal baths are not just about cleanliness; they offer therapeutic benefits, allowing the body to absorb herbs through the skin.

Preparing Herbal Baths

- Fill a muslin bag with herbs and hang it under the tap, letting hot water run through it as the bath fills.

- Alternatively, make a strong herbal infusion, strain it, and add it to the bathwater.

Incorporating these herbal preparations into your life aligns with the principles of holistic wellness. It's not just about treating symptoms but about fostering a deeper connection with nature and our bodies. Each method offers a unique way to harness the healing power of plants, reminding us that sometimes, the most effective remedies are the ones provided by nature itself.

Safe Storage and Shelf Life of Herbal Remedies

Herbal remedies, derived from the bounty of nature, have been a cornerstone of all-rounded health and wellness practices for centuries. Their ability to promote healing and well-being hinges significantly on how they are stored and their shelf life. Proper storage not only extends the efficacy of these natural treasures but also ensures their safety for use.

Understanding Herbal Remedies

Before delving into storage and shelf life, it's essential to appreciate what herbal remedies are. These are preparations made from plant materials – leaves, stems, roots, seeds, or flowers – used to prevent, alleviate, or cure ailments. They come in various forms like teas, tinctures, capsules, powders, and oils. Each form has unique storage requirements and shelf life considerations.

The Importance of Proper Storage

Why is storage so crucial for herbal remedies? Herbs, like any organic material, are susceptible to environmental factors. Exposure to light, heat, moisture, and air can degrade their quality, potency, and safety. Proper storage conditions preserve their therapeutic properties and prevent contamination or spoilage.

Best Practices for Storage

1. **Darkness and Light Sensitivity**: Many herbs and their preparations are sensitive to light, especially direct sunlight, which can cause them to degrade. Storing them in dark, amber-colored glass containers helps protect them from light exposure.

2. **Temperature Control**: Excessive heat can spoil herbal remedies by accelerating chemical degradation. It's recommended to store them in a cool, dry place, preferably at room temperature.

3. **Moisture and Air Exposure**: Herbs need to be kept dry as moisture can lead to mold growth and spoilage. Airtight containers are crucial to prevent exposure to air, which can lead to oxidation and loss of potency.

4. **Safe Containers**: The material of the container also matters. Glass is generally preferable over plastic, as it is inert and doesn't interact with the herbs. If plastic must be used, ensure it's food-grade quality.

Factors Affecting Shelf Life

Several factors determine how long your herbal remedies will remain effective:

1. **Type of Herb**: Some herbs are more resilient than others. For instance, roots and barks usually last longer than leaves and flowers.

2. **Form of the Remedy**: Dried herbs, tinctures, and oils have different shelf lives. Generally, tinctures and oils last longer than dried herbs.

3. **Quality at Time of Preparation**: The initial quality of the herb, including how it was grown, harvested, and processed, plays a significant role in its shelf life.

4. **Additives and Preservatives**: Some preparations include natural preservatives like alcohol in tinctures, which can extend shelf life.

Estimating Shelf Life

While it's challenging to assign a definitive shelf life to each herbal remedy due to varying factors, here are general guidelines:

1. **Dried Herbs**: Properly stored, dried herbs can last up to two years. Their potency diminishes over time, so it's vital to observe any changes in color, smell, or texture.

2. **Tinctures**: Alcohol-based tinctures have a longer shelf life, often several years, due to the preserving nature of alcohol.

3. **Herbal Oils**: These can vary, but typically last around one year. If they contain antioxidants or are refrigerated, they may last longer.

4. **Capsules and Powders**: They generally last about two years but check for any signs of spoilage like dampness or discoloration.

Signs of Degradation

Recognizing when an herbal remedy has gone bad is crucial. Look for signs like:

- Mold or mildew growth

- Unpleasant or rancid odor

- Discoloration or change in texture

- Loss of aroma in dried herbs

Tips for Extending Shelf Life

1. **Labeling**: Always label containers with the date of packaging or purchase and the expected shelf life.

2. **Quantity**: Store in quantities that you will use within the expected shelf life.

3. **Regular Checks**: Periodically check your stored remedies for any signs of spoilage.

4. **Special Care for Oils and Tinctures**: Keep oils in cool places and tinctures in dark bottles away from direct light.

The effective use of herbal remedies not only lies in their selection but also in how they are stored and maintained. By understanding and implementing proper storage techniques and being mindful of their shelf life, one can ensure that these natural gifts retain their healing properties, contributing to a complete approach to health and wellness.

CHAPTER 3: 101 HERBAL REMEDIES YOU SHOULD KNOW AND HOW TO USE THEM

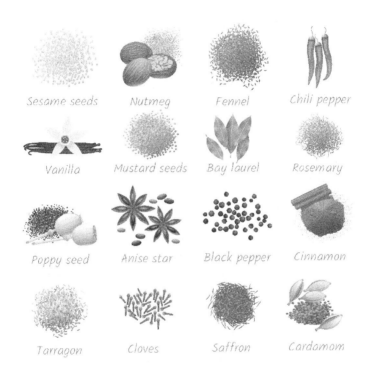

Sesame seeds	Nutmeg	Fennel	Chili pepper
Vanilla	Mustard seeds	Bay laurel	Rosemary
Poppy seed	Anise star	Black pepper	Cinnamon
Tarragon	Cloves	Saffron	Cardamom

1. **Aloe Vera**

   - Origin: Native to North Africa, Southern Europe, and the Canary Islands.

   - Uses: Soothing skin irritations, burns, and aiding digestion.

- Benefits: Moisturizes skin, heals wounds, and relieves heartburn.

- How to Use: Apply gel topically for skin issues; drink juice for digestive health.

- Interesting Fact: Known as the "plant of immortality" in ancient Egypt.

- Safety: Topical use is generally safe; oral use may have laxative effects.

2. **Arnica**

- Origin: Native to Europe and Siberia, found in grassy, alpine meadows.

- Uses: Treating bruises, sprains, and muscle soreness.

- Benefits: Anti-inflammatory properties, and pain relief.

- How to Use: Apply as a cream or gel to affected areas (not on broken skin).

- Interesting Fact: Used by mountain guides in the Swiss Alps for injuries.

- Safety: Toxic when ingested; only use topically.

3. **Ashwagandha**

- Origin: Native to India and North Africa.

- Uses: Reducing stress and anxiety, improving energy levels.

- Benefits: Adaptogenic properties, enhances vitality and concentration.

- How to Use: Consumed as a powder, pill, or extract.

- Interesting Fact: Known as 'Indian Ginseng' for its restorative benefits.

- Safety: Generally safe; may interact with certain medications.

4. **Astragalus**

- Origin: Traditional Chinese medicine, from a type of legume or bean.

- Uses: Boosting the immune system.

- Benefits: Antioxidant effects, supports cardiovascular health.

- How to Use: Consumed as a supplement, extract, or tea.

- Interesting Fact: Used in Chinese medicine for over 2,000 years.

- Safety: Avoid if you have autoimmune diseases or are on immune-suppressants.

5. **Basil**

- Origin: Native to tropical regions from Central Africa to Southeast Asia.

- Uses: Culinary and medicinal, particularly for its essential oil.

- Benefits: Reduces inflammation, and fights bacteria.

- How to Use: Fresh in cooking, or as an essential oil.

- Interesting Fact: Revered as a sacred herb in Hinduism.

- Safety: Generally safe; essential oil should be diluted.

6. **Black Cohosh**

- Origin: Native to North America.

- Uses: Alleviating menopause symptoms like hot flashes and mood swings.

- Benefits: Mimics estrogen, which can decrease menopause symptoms.

- How to Use: Taken as a supplement in capsule or liquid form.

- Interesting Fact: Known as a "fairy candle" due to its tall white flowers.

- Safety: May cause liver issues; not recommended for pregnant women.

7. **Burdock Root**

- Origin: Europe and Asia.

- Uses: Detoxifying the body, and improving skin health.

- Benefits: Contains antioxidants; aids in purifying blood.

- How to Use: Eaten as a vegetable, taken as a supplement, or used as tea.

- Interesting Fact: Burdock is a staple in Japanese cuisine, known as "gobo".

- Safety: Generally safe; may cause allergic reactions in some.

8. **Calendula**

- Origin: Mediterranean region.
- Uses: Healing wounds, reducing inflammation.
- Benefits: Antifungal, anti-inflammatory, and antibacterial properties.
- How to Use: Applied topically as a cream or ointment.
- Interesting Fact: Used in the American Civil War for wound treatment.
- Safety: Avoid during pregnancy; may cause an allergic reaction in rare cases.

9. **Cardamom**

- Origin: Native to the Indian subcontinent and Indonesia.
- Uses: Digestive aid, relieving nausea, and combating bad breath.

- Benefits: Contains antioxidants, and supports digestive health.

- How to Use: Used in cooking or chewed as a fresh pod.

- Interesting Fact: Known as the "Queen of Spices" in India.

- Safety: Generally safe; excessive consumption may lead to gallstone issues.

10. **Catnip**

- Origin: Native to Europe and Asia, naturalized in North America.

- Uses: Reducing stress, aiding sleep, and soothing digestive issues.

- Benefits: Relaxant effects, mild sedative properties.

- How to Use: Consumed as tea or in capsule form.

- Interesting Fact: Famous for its stimulating effect on cats.

- Safety: Generally safe; avoid if pregnant or breastfeeding.

11. Cayenne

- Origin: Native to the Americas.

- Uses: Pain relief, boosting metabolism.

- Benefits: Anti-inflammatory, aids in digestion, improves circulation.

- How to Use: Added to food, taken as a capsule, or used in creams.

- Historical Info: Used in Native American medicine for various ailments.

- Safety: May irritate if applied topically; stomach discomfort if ingested in large amounts.

12. Chamomile

- Origin: Europe and Western Asia.

- Uses: Inducing sleep, soothing digestion.

- Benefits: Anti-inflammatory, relaxant, helps with anxiety.

- How to Use: Commonly consumed as tea.

- Historical Info: Ancient Egyptians used it for its healing properties.
- Safety: Rarely, allergic reactions; avoid if allergic to ragweed.

13. **Chaste Tree Berry**

- Origin: Mediterranean region.
- Uses: Balancing hormones, especially in women.
- Benefits: Eases menstrual symptoms, and may aid in fertility.
- How to Use: Taken as a supplement.
- Historical Info: Known as the "women's herb" in ancient times.
- Safety: Not for pregnant or breastfeeding women; may interact with hormonal medications.

14. **Cinnamon**

- Origin: Sri Lanka, India.
- Uses: Blood sugar control, anti-inflammatory.
- Benefits: Antioxidant, antimicrobial, may lower cholesterol.

- How to Use: Added to food and drinks.
- Historical Info: Valued in ancient Egypt for its rarity and healing properties.
- Safety: High doses can be toxic; coumarin in Cassia cinnamon can be harmful in large amounts.

15. **Clove**

- Origin: Indonesia.
- Uses: Relieving toothache, antibacterial.
- Benefits: Antioxidants, may improve liver health.
- How to Use: Applied topically for pain relief; used in cooking.
- Historical Info: Widely used in traditional Chinese and Ayurvedic medicine.
- Safety: May irritate skin; excessive use can cause liver damage.

16. **Comfrey**

- Origin: Europe.

- Uses: Wound healing, anti-inflammatory.

- Benefits: Accelerates skin healing, and reduces inflammation.

- How to Use: As a cream or poultice for external use.

- Historical Info: Known as "knitbone" in folk medicine.

- Safety: Contains pyrrolizidine alkaloids, which can be toxic; not for internal use or open wounds.

17. Cranberry

- Origin: North America.

- Uses: Preventing urinary tract infections.

- Benefits: Contains proanthocyanidins that prevent bacteria adherence.

- How to Use: Consumed as juice or supplements.

- Historical Info: Native Americans used it as a treatment for bladder and kidney diseases.

- Safety: Generally safe; excessive consumption can lead to stomach upset.

18. **Dandelion**

- Origin: Eurasia.

- Uses: Liver support, and digestive aid.

- Benefits: Diuretic, supports liver function, rich in vitamins.

- How to Use: Leaves and roots are used in teas, salads, or supplements.

- Historical Info: Used in traditional medicine for centuries for liver ailments.

- Safety: Generally safe; possible allergic reactions.

19. **Dill**

- Origin: Eastern Mediterranean, Western Asia.

- Uses: Digestive aid, bad breath remedy.

- Benefits: Antioxidant, antibacterial, aids in digestion.

- How to Use: Used in cooking or as a tea.

- Historical Info: Ancient Greeks and Romans used it for its medicinal properties.

- Safety: Generally safe; can cause skin irritation if allergic.

20. Echinacea

- Origin: North America.

- Uses: Boosting the immune system.

- Benefits: May reduce cold symptoms and duration.

- How to Use: Taken as a tea, tincture, or capsule.

- Historical Info: Widely used by Native Americans for various conditions.

- Safety: May cause allergic reactions, especially in those allergic to daisies.

21. Elderberry

- Origin: Europe, North America, and parts of Asia.

- Uses: Cold and flu relief.

- Benefits: High in vitamins and antioxidants, supports the immune system.

- How to Use: Commonly taken as syrup or in capsules.

- Historical Info: Used in folk medicine for centuries; believed to ward off evil in some cultures.

- Safety: Raw berries are toxic; only cooked berries should be used.

22. Eucalyptus

- Origin: Australia.

- Uses: Treating respiratory issues, decongestant.

- Benefits: Antimicrobial, helps ease coughs and congestion.

- How to Use: Inhaled as an essential oil or used in chest rubs.

- Historical Info: Long used by Indigenous Australians for healing wounds.

- Safety: Essential oil can be toxic if ingested; not for use on the skin of young children.

23. Evening Primrose Oil

- Origin: North America and parts of Europe.

- Uses: Skin health, hormonal balance.

- Benefits: Contains GLA (gamma-linolenic acid), beneficial for skin conditions and PMS.

- How to Use: Taken as an oil or in capsules.

- Historical Info: Native Americans used the whole plant for bruises and digestive issues.

- Safety: May interact with blood thinners; can cause mild side effects like headache.

24. Fennel

- Origin: Mediterranean.

- Uses: Digestive aid, gas relief.

- Benefits: Antispasmodic, aids in digestion, supports breastfeeding.

- How to Use: Seeds are used in cooking or as tea.

- Historical Info: Ancient Egyptians and Romans regarded it for its medicinal properties.

- Safety: Generally safe; excessive doses can be toxic.

25. **Fenugreek**

- Origin: Mediterranean region, Southern Europe, and Western Asia.

- Uses: Blood sugar regulation, lactation aid.

- Benefits: Helps with diabetes management, and increases milk production in breastfeeding.

- How to Use: Seeds are used in cooking or as supplements.

- Historical Info: Used in ancient Egyptian, Greek, and Roman medicine.

- Safety: Can cause mild gastrointestinal symptoms; may interact with blood sugar medications.

26. **Feverfew**

- Origin: Southeastern Europe.

- Uses: Migraine and headache relief.

- Benefits: Anti-inflammatory properties, reduce migraine frequency.

- How to Use: Consumed as tea or in capsules.

- Historical Info: Used since ancient times for fever, headaches, and as an anti-inflammatory.

- Safety: This can cause mouth ulcers and digestive issues; withdrawal can lead to rebound headaches.

27. **Flaxseed**

- Origin: Middle East.

- Uses: Digestive health, cholesterol management.

- Benefits: High in fiber, omega-3 fatty acids, lignans.

- How to Use: Ground seeds added to food, or taken as oil.

- Historical Info: Used since ancient times, known for its health benefits in the Roman Empire.

- Safety: Generally safe; large doses can cause bowel obstruction.

28. **Garlic**

- Origin: Central Asia.

- Uses: Cardiovascular health, immune support.

- Benefits: Antimicrobial, reduces blood pressure and cholesterol.

- How to Use: Consumed raw or cooked; available in supplement form.

- Historical Info: Used in ancient civilizations for its medicinal properties and as a performance enhancer.

- Safety: Generally safe; can cause bad breath, digestive issues, and interfere with blood thinners.

29. Ginger

- Origin: Southeast Asia.

- Uses: Nausea relief, anti-inflammatory.

- Benefits: Digestive aid, reduces nausea, anti-inflammatory properties.

- How to Use: Consumed fresh, dried, or as tea; also available in supplements.

- Historical Info: Long history of use in various traditional medicines, including Ayurveda.

- Safety: Generally safe; high doses can cause heartburn and diarrhea.

30. Ginkgo Biloba

- Origin: China.

- Uses: Cognitive function, circulation.

- Benefits: Antioxidant, improves blood flow, enhances brain health.

- How to Use: Taken as an extract in capsules or tablets.

- Historical Info: One of the oldest living tree species, used for millennia in Chinese medicine.

- Safety: Can interact with blood thinners; may cause headache, and dizziness.

31.**Ginseng**

- Origin: Native to East Asia and North America.

- Uses: Traditionally used to boost energy and reduce stress.

- Benefits: Enhances physical and mental endurance, and improves concentration.

- How to Use: Consumed as tea, capsules, or extracts.

- Historical/Cultural Info: Revered in traditional Chinese medicine for centuries.

- Safety/Side Effects: Can cause insomnia, and high blood pressure in high doses.

32. Goldenrod

- Origin: Europe and parts of Asia and North America.

- Uses: Treats urinary tract infections, and reduces inflammation.

- Benefits: Supports urinary tract health, and acts as an anti-inflammatory agent.

- How to Use: Tea or tincture.

- Historical/Cultural Info: Used in traditional medicine for kidney and bladder ailments.

- Safety/Side Effects: Allergies in sensitive individuals.

33. Goldenseal

- Origin: North America.

- Uses: Digestive and respiratory system support.

- Benefits: Antibacterial, helps soothe an upset stomach.

- How to Use: Capsules, tea, or liquid extracts.

- Historical/Cultural Info: Used by Native Americans for various health issues.

- Safety/Side Effects: Not recommended during pregnancy or for long-term use.

34. Gotu Kola

- Origin: Asia.

- Uses: Wound healing, cognitive enhancement.

- Benefits: Promotes skin healing, and improves memory and circulation.

- How to Use: Tea, capsules, or topical ointments.

- Historical/Cultural Info: A staple in Ayurvedic and traditional Chinese medicine.

- Safety/Side Effects: This may cause headaches or dizziness in high doses.

35. Grape Seed Extract

- Origin: Extracted from the seeds of grapes.

- Uses: Antioxidant and cardiovascular support.

- Benefits: Protects against oxidative stress, and supports heart health.

- How to Use: Usually taken in capsule form.

- Historical/Cultural Info: Evolved from traditional wine cultures.

- Safety/Side Effects: Generally safe, may interfere with blood thinners.

36. Green Tea

- Origin: East Asia.

- Uses: Antioxidant properties, boosts metabolism.

- Benefits: May reduce the risk of heart disease, and aid weight loss.

- How to Use: As a beverage or in extract form.

- Historical/Cultural Info: Centuries-old beverage, integral to many Asian cultures.

- Safety/Side Effects: Excessive consumption can cause insomnia due to caffeine.

37.Hawthorn Berry

- Origin: Europe, North America, and Asia.

- Uses: Heart health, blood pressure management.

- Benefits: Improves cardiac function, and regulates blood pressure.

- How to Use: Tea, capsules, or liquid extract.

- Historical/Cultural Info: Long history in European herbal medicine.

- Safety/Side Effects: Can interact with heart medications.

38.Hibiscus

- Origin: Warm temperate, subtropical, and tropical regions.

- Uses: Blood pressure management, antioxidant.

- Benefits: Lowers blood pressure, rich in vitamin C.

- How to Use: Commonly consumed as tea.

- Historical/Cultural Info: Used in traditional medicine and as a natural dye.

- Safety/Side Effects: Can lower blood pressure significantly.

39. **Holy Basil**

- Origin: Native to India.

- Uses: Stress relief, anti-inflammatory.

- Benefits: Adaptogenic properties, boosts immunity.

- How to Use: Tea, fresh leaves, or supplements.

- Historical/Cultural Info: Considered a sacred plant in Hindu belief.

- Safety/Side Effects: Avoid during pregnancy or if trying to conceive.

40. Hops

- Origin: Europe, Western Asia, and North America.

- Uses: Sleep aid, anxiety, and stress relief.

- Benefits: Sedative effects, can improve sleep quality.

- How to Use: In teas, extracts, or as a supplement.

- Historical/Cultural Info: Best known for use in brewing beer.

- Safety/Side Effects: This may cause drowsiness.

41. Horehound

- Origin: Europe, North Africa, and parts of Asia.

- Uses: Respiratory health and digestion.

- Benefits: Helps with coughs and aids digestion.

- How to Use: Typically used in teas, lozenges, or syrups.

- Historical/Cultural Info: An ancient remedy, mentioned in old texts for its medicinal properties.

- Safety/Side Effects: This should be avoided during pregnancy.

42. Horse Chestnut

- Origin: Balkans; widely cultivated elsewhere.

- Uses: Improves vein health, and reduces inflammation.

- Benefits: Treats varicose veins and hemorrhoids.

- How to Use: Capsules, creams, or extracts.

- Historical/Cultural Info: Long used in Europe for circulatory health.

- Safety/Side Effects: Raw seeds are toxic; only processed forms should be used.

43. Horsetail

- Origin: Europe, Asia, North America, and the Middle East.

- Uses: Bone and hair health.

- Benefits: Source of silica for strong bones and nails.

- How to Use: Tea or supplements.

- Historical/Cultural Info: Used by ancient Romans and Greeks for health benefits.

- Safety/Side Effects: Long-term use is not recommended; can cause thiamine deficiency.

44. Hyssop

- Origin: Southern Europe, Middle East.

- Uses: Respiratory health and digestion.

- Benefits: Helps relieve congestion and aids digestion.

- How to Use: As a tea or in essential oil form.

- Historical/Cultural Info: Mentioned in the Bible and used historically in ritual cleansing.

- Safety/Side Effects: Should be avoided by pregnant women and those with epilepsy.

45. Jasmine

- Origin: Asia, especially China and India.

- Uses: Stress relief and antioxidant properties.

- Benefits: Soothes the nervous system, and promotes relaxation.

- How to Use: Commonly consumed as tea.

- Historical/Cultural Info: Widely used in aromatherapy and traditional ceremonies.

- Safety/Side Effects: Generally safe; excessive consumption can cause discomfort.

46. Juniper Berry

- Origin: Northern Hemisphere.

- Uses: Digestive aid and detoxification.

- Benefits: Supports digestion, and has diuretic properties.

- How to Use: In tea or as an essential oil.

- Historical/Cultural Info: Used historically for medicinal and culinary purposes.

- Safety/Side Effects: Not recommended for pregnant women or those with kidney issues.

47. Kava Kava

- Origin: South Pacific Islands.

- Uses: Anxiety relief and as a sleep aid.

- Benefits: Sedative and euphoric effects.

- How to Use: Consumed as a drink, extract, or in capsule form.

- Historical/Cultural Info: An important part of Pacific Islander cultural rituals.

- Safety/Side Effects: Can affect liver function; should be used with caution.

48. Krill Oil

- Origin: Extracted from Antarctic krill.

- Uses: Source of Omega-3 fatty acids, supports heart health.

- Benefits: Reduces inflammation, and supports cardiovascular and brain health.

- How to Use: Available in soft gel capsules.

- Historical/Cultural Info: Gained popularity as an alternative to fish oil.

- Safety/Side Effects: May interact with anticoagulant medications.

49. Lavender

- Origin: Mediterranean region.

- Uses: Relaxation and skin health.

- Benefits: Calming effect, promotes skin healing.

- How to Use: Essential oil for aromatherapy or topical use; dried flowers for tea.

- Historical/Cultural Info: Used since ancient times for its fragrance and medicinal properties.

- Safety/Side Effects: Generally safe; oral ingestion in large amounts can be harmful.

50. Lemon Balm

- Origin: Europe, Central Asia.

- Uses: Stress relief and digestive health.

- Benefits: Calms the mind, and soothes digestive issues.

- How to Use: Commonly used in teas or as an essential oil.

- Historical/Cultural Info: Historically used to uplift spirits and help with digestion.

- Safety/Side Effects: Generally safe, may interact with thyroid medications.

51. Lemongrass

- Origin: Native to tropical regions such as India, Africa, and Southeast Asia.

- Uses: Aids in digestion, relieves stress, and acts as a natural insect repellent.

- Benefits: Contains antioxidants, has antimicrobial properties, and can help reduce anxiety.

- How to Use: Commonly used in teas, cooking, and as an essential oil.

- Interesting Fact: In traditional Brazilian medicine, it's used for its sedative effects.

- Safety: Generally safe, but may cause allergies in sensitive individuals.

52. Licorice Root

- Origin: Native to Southern Europe and parts of Asia.

- Uses: Soothes gastrointestinal problems, treats respiratory issues, and relieves sore throat.

- Benefits: Anti-inflammatory and immune-boosting properties.

- How to Use: Consumed as tea, chewed as a root, or taken as a supplement.

- Interesting Fact: It's been used in traditional Chinese medicine for thousands of years.

- Safety: Long-term use can lead to high blood pressure and low potassium levels.

53.**Maca Root**

- Origin: Native to the high Andes of Peru.

- Uses: Enhances energy, improves mood, and balances hormones.

- Benefits: Rich in vitamins and minerals; supports sexual health.

- How to Use: Typically taken in powder form or as a supplement.

- Interesting Fact: Known as "Peruvian ginseng" despite having no botanical relation to ginseng.

- Safety: Generally safe, but pregnant women should consult a doctor before use.

54.**Marshmallow Root**

- Origin: Europe, Western Asia, and North Africa.

- Uses: Soothes respiratory and digestive systems.

- Benefits: Contains mucilage which helps coat and calm mucous membranes.

- How to Use: Often consumed as a tea or in lozenge form.

- Interesting Fact: Historically used in ancient Egyptian confections.

- Safety: Safe for most people, but diabetic patients should monitor blood sugar levels.

55. Milk Thistle

- Origin: Native to Mediterranean countries.

- Uses: Protects the liver, and promotes liver regeneration.

- Benefits: High in antioxidants, particularly silymarin.

- How to Use: Taken as a supplement or as tea.

- Interesting Fact: Used in Europe as a remedy for liver problems for over 2,000 years.

- Safety: Generally safe; rare side effects include gastrointestinal upset.

56. Mint

- Origin: Native to Europe and Asia.

- Uses: Aids digestion, freshens breath, and relieves headaches.

- Benefits: Contains menthol, which has a cooling effect and can help relieve pain.

- How to Use: Consumed in teas, used in cooking, or inhaled as essential oil.

- Interesting Fact: Ancient Greeks used mint in baths and as a cleaning agent.

- Safety: May cause heartburn in some people.

57. Motherwort

- Origin: Native to Eurasia.

- Uses: Supports heart health and helps alleviate menstrual cramps.

- Benefits: Calming effects, good for reducing heart palpitations and anxiety.

- How to Use: Typically consumed as tea or tincture.

- Interesting Fact: Its name is derived from its traditional use in ancient Greek and Roman medicine as a remedy for pregnant women.

- Safety: Should not be used during pregnancy except under medical supervision.

58. Mullein

- Origin: Native to Europe, North Africa, and Asia.

- Uses: Treats respiratory ailments and reduces inflammation.

- Benefits: Soothes the respiratory tract and helps expel mucus.

- How to Use: Consumed as a tea, inhaled as steam, or applied topically.

- Interesting Fact: During the Middle Ages, it was used to ward off evil spirits.

- Safety: Generally safe, but seeds are toxic and should not be consumed.

59. Nettle

- Origin: Widely found in Europe, Asia, and North America.

- Uses: Alleviates allergies, and provides nutritional support.

- Benefits: Rich in nutrients, anti-inflammatory, and antihistamine properties.

- How to Use: Consumed as tea, in soups, or as a cooked green.

- Interesting Fact: Nettle fibers were used to make cloth in ancient times.

- Safety: May cause skin irritation upon contact; cooking or drying neutralizes the stinging hairs.

60. Oat Straw

- Origin: Derived from the same plant as oatmeal, native to Northern Europe.

- Uses: Enhances mood, supports the nervous system, and relieves stress.

- Benefits: Rich in vitamins and minerals, particularly good for skin health.

- How to Use: Consumed as a tea or in baths.

- Interesting Fact: Traditionally used as a remedy to support brain health in medieval Europe.

- Safety: Very safe, but people with celiac disease should ensure it's gluten-free.

61.**Olive Leaf**

- Origin: Mediterranean region.

- Uses: Boosts the immune system, and improves cardiovascular health.

- Benefits: Rich in antioxidants and has anti-inflammatory properties.

- How to Use: Taken as a supplement or tea.

- Interesting Fact: Olive leaf has been used medicinally in various cultures for centuries.

- Safety: Generally safe but can lower blood pressure; those on blood pressure medication should consult a doctor.

62. Oregano

- Origin: Native to Western and Southwestern Eurasia and the Mediterranean region.

- Uses: Antioxidant support, antibacterial and anti-inflammatory effects.

- Benefits: Contains compounds like thymol and carvacrol which offer health benefits.

- How to Use: Used in cooking or as oil.

- Interesting Fact: Oregano was commonly used by the ancient Greeks for medicinal purposes.

- Safety: Generally safe when consumed in food; oregano oil should be diluted before topical use.

63. Parsley

- Origin: Mediterranean region.

- Uses: Supports digestion and detoxification.

- Benefits: Rich in vitamins A, C, and K, and contains antioxidants.

- How to Use: Commonly used in cooking as a garnish and flavor enhancer.

- Interesting Fact: In ancient times, parsley wreaths were used to ward off drunkenness.

- Safety: Safe in food amounts; large medicinal amounts should be avoided during pregnancy.

64. Passionflower

- Origin: Native to the southeastern United States, Central and South America.

- Uses: Relieves anxiety and improves sleep.

- Benefits: Contains compounds that have calming effects.

- How to Use: Consumed as tea or in supplement form.

- Interesting Fact: Traditionally used by Native Americans to treat a variety of conditions.

- Safety: Generally safe; may cause drowsiness.

65. Pau d'Arco

- Origin: South America.

- Uses: Reduces inflammation and fights fungal infections.

- Benefits: Contains naphthoquinones, which have antifungal and anti-inflammatory properties.

- How to Use: Typically consumed as a tea or in supplement form.

- Interesting Fact: Indigenous tribes in South America have used it for its healing properties for centuries.

- Safety: Large doses can be toxic; not recommended during pregnancy.

66. Peppermint

- Origin: Europe and the Middle East.

- Uses: Aids digestion and relieves headaches.

- Benefits: Menthol provides a cooling sensation and can help ease pain.

- How to Use: Consumed as tea, used in aromatherapy, or applied topically.

- Interesting Fact: Peppermint has been used medicinally since ancient Egyptian times.

- Safety: Generally safe; peppermint oil should not be applied to the face of infants or small children.

67. Plantain Leaf

- Origin: Europe and Asia.

- Uses: Skin healing and anti-inflammatory.

- Benefits: Contains allantoin, which promotes wound healing.

- How to Use: Applied topically as a poultice or cream.

- Interesting Fact: Known as the "healing plant" in some traditional cultures.

- Safety: Generally safe when used on the skin.

68. Red Clover

- Origin: Europe, Western Asia, and Northwest Africa.

- Uses: Improves blood flow and relieves menopause symptoms.

- Benefits: Contains isoflavones, which mimic estrogen.

- How to Use: Consumed as tea or in supplement form.

- Interesting Fact: Traditionally used in folk medicine as a purifying herb.

- Safety: May interact with hormonal medications; not recommended for those with hormone-sensitive conditions.

69. Red Raspberry Leaf

- Origin: Native to Europe and parts of Asia.

- Uses: Supports women's health and aids digestion.

- Benefits: Rich in vitamins and minerals, especially beneficial during pregnancy.

- How to Use: Commonly consumed as tea.

- Interesting Fact: Often referred to as a "woman's herb" for its benefits to the female reproductive system.

- Safety: Generally considered safe, particularly popular among pregnant women, though consultation with a healthcare provider is advised.

70. **Reishi Mushroom**

- Origin: East Asia.

- Uses: Boosts the immune system and relieves stress.

- Benefits: Known as the "mushroom of immortality," it has adaptogenic properties.

- How to Use: Taken as a supplement or in tea form.

- Interesting Fact: Has been a staple in Eastern medicine for over 2,000 years.

- Safety: Generally safe, but can interact with certain medications like blood thinners.

71. **Rhodiola Rosea**

- Origin: Native to the Arctic regions of Europe, Asia, and North America.

- Uses: Stress relief and boosting energy.

- Benefits: Helps the body adapt to stress, and improves mental performance and physical stamina.

- How to Use: Commonly taken as a supplement or extract.

- Interesting Fact: Known as a "golden root" or "Arctic root" in traditional medicine.

- Safety: Generally safe but can cause dizziness and dry mouth in some.

72. **Rose Hips**

- Origin: Derived from the fruit of the rose plant.

- Uses: As a vitamin C source and for immune support.

- Benefits: High in antioxidants and may help reduce joint pain.

- How to Use: Consumed as tea, jam, jelly, or supplements.

- Interesting Fact: Used during World War II when citrus fruits were scarce.

- Safety: Usually safe, but excessive consumption can cause stomach upset.

73. **Rosemary**

- Origin: Mediterranean region.

- Uses: For cognitive function and aiding digestion.

- Benefits: Enhances memory and concentration, and has anti-inflammatory properties.

- How to Use: Used in cooking, as a tea, or as an essential oil.

- Interesting Fact: In folklore, rosemary is known to improve memory.

- Safety: Safe in culinary amounts; large doses can cause vomiting and spasms.

74.**Sage**

- Origin: Mediterranean region.

- Uses: For cognitive health and digestion.

- Benefits: Antioxidant properties and may alleviate menopause symptoms.

- How to Use: Used in cooking, as tea, or as a supplement.

- Interesting Fact: Historically used for warding off evil and snakebites.

- Safety: Generally safe but not recommended in high doses or for pregnant women.

75.**Sarsaparilla**

- Origin: Native to South America, Jamaica, the Caribbean, Mexico, Honduras, and the West Indies.

- Uses: Skin health and detoxification.

- Benefits: Anti-inflammatory properties and can purify the blood.

- How to Use: Often taken as a tea or supplement.

- Interesting Fact: Once popular as the main flavoring for root beer.

- Safety: Generally safe but can interact with certain medications.

76. Saw Palmetto

- Origin: Southeastern United States.

- Uses: Prostate health and hormonal balance.

- Benefits: May improve urinary function and reduce inflammation.

- How to Use: Usually taken as a capsule or liquid extract.

- Interesting Fact: Traditionally used by Native Americans for urinary and reproductive problems.

- Safety: Well-tolerated, but can cause mild side effects like stomach discomfort.

77. Schisandra Berry

- Origin: Native to East Asia.

- Uses: Liver support and stress relief.

- Benefits: Boosts liver function and improves stress resistance.

- How to Use: Consumed as dried berries, tea, or supplements.

- Interesting Fact: Known as a "five-flavor berry" due to its complex taste.

- Safety: Generally safe; rare side effects include heartburn and upset stomach.

78. Senna Leaf

- Origin: Native to North Africa and the Middle East.

- Uses: As a natural laxative and digestive aid.

- Benefits: Effective for short-term relief of constipation.

- How to Use: Taken as tea, capsules, or tablets.

- Interesting Fact: Has been used for centuries in traditional Arabian medicine.

- Safety: Short-term use is safe; long-term use can lead to dependency.

79. **Shatavari**

- Origin: India and the Himalayas.

- Uses: Women's health and reproductive support.

- Benefits: May help with fertility, menstrual cycles, and menopausal symptoms.

- How to Use: Commonly taken as a powder or tablet.

- Interesting Fact: Its name means "a woman with a hundred husbands" in Sanskrit.

- Safety: Generally safe; possible side effects include allergic reactions.

80. **Shepherd's Purse**

- Origin: Europe and parts of Asia.

- Uses: Menstrual health and improving circulation.

- Benefits: May help reduce bleeding and improve blood clotting.

- How to Use: Often used as a tea or tincture.

- Interesting Fact: Used in traditional Chinese medicine to stop bleeding.

- Safety: Generally safe, but not recommended for pregnant women.

81. Skullcap

- Origin: Native to North America.

- Uses: Anxiety relief and sleep aid.

- Benefits: Promotes relaxation and can aid in treating insomnia.

- How to Use: Often consumed as tea or as a supplement.

- Interesting Fact: Historically used by Native Americans for menstrual irregularities and nervous conditions.

- Safety: Generally safe in moderate amounts; high doses can cause confusion and seizures.

82. Slippery Elm

- Origin: Central and Eastern United States.

- Uses: Digestive health and sore throat relief.

- Benefits: Soothes the digestive tract and can relieve coughs.

- How to Use: As a lozenge, tea, or supplement.

- Interesting Fact: The inner bark was used as survival food in American history.

- Safety: Generally safe; possible allergic reactions in sensitive individuals.

83. Spearmint

- Origin: Europe and Asia.

- Uses: Digestive health and hormone balance.

- Benefits: Can help with digestion and may reduce hirsutism in women.

- How to Use: Commonly used as tea or added to food.

- Interesting Fact: Spearmint has been used for centuries in traditional medicines.

- Safety: Safe in food amounts; large medicinal amounts might cause liver damage.

84. St. John's Wort

- Origin: Europe and Asia, now worldwide.

- Uses: Mood enhancement and sleep aid.

- Benefits: Commonly used for depression and may improve sleep quality.

- How to Use: Typically taken as a supplement or tea.

- Interesting Fact: Its name derives from its traditional flowering and harvesting on St John's Day, 24 June.

- Safety: Can interact with numerous medications; can cause photosensitivity.

85. Stevia

- Origin: South America.

- Uses: As a natural sweetener and for blood sugar regulation.

- Benefits: Zero-calorie sweetener, may help in managing diabetes.

- How to Use: Used as a sugar substitute in foods and beverages.

- Interesting Fact: The Guaraní peoples of South America have used stevia for centuries.

- Safety: Generally recognized as safe; some people might experience bloating or nausea.

86. Thyme

- Origin: Southern Europe and the Mediterranean.

- Uses: Respiratory health and antibacterial effects.

- Benefits: Can alleviate cough and has strong antimicrobial properties.

- How to Use: Used in cooking, as a tea, or essential oil.

- Interesting Fact: Thyme was used in embalming practices in ancient Egypt.

- Safety: Safe in food amounts; excessive use can disrupt the hormonal balance.

87. **Triphala**

- Origin: Traditional Ayurvedic medicine from India.

- Uses: Digestive aid and detoxification.

- Benefits: Promotes bowel health and can aid in body detoxification.

- How to Use: Commonly taken as a supplement or powder.

- Interesting Fact: Triphala means "three fruits," which are Amalaki, Bibhitaki, and Haritaki.

- Safety: Generally safe; overuse can lead to gastrointestinal issues.

88. Turmeric

- Origin: Southeast Asia and the Indian subcontinent.

- Uses: Anti-inflammatory and antioxidant.

- Benefits: Reduces inflammation, beneficial for joint health and cognitive function.

- How to Use: Used in cooking, as supplements, or in beverages like "golden milk."

- Interesting Fact: Integral to Ayurvedic medicine as a cleansing herb.

- Safety: Generally safe; high doses can cause stomach upset and thin blood.

89. Uva Ursi

- Origin: Northern hemisphere's colder regions.

- Uses: Urinary tract health and anti-inflammatory.

- Benefits: Helps in treating urinary tract infections and reduces inflammation.

- How to Use: Typically as a tea or supplement.

- Interesting Fact: Its leaves have been used in traditional medicine since the 2nd century.

- Safety: Short-term use is recommended; long-term use can be harmful.

90. **Valerian Root**

- Origin: Europe and parts of Asia.

- Uses: Sleep aid and anxiety relief.

- Benefits: Promotes relaxation and improves sleep quality.

- How to Use: As tea, tincture, or supplement.

- Interesting Fact: Known as "nature's Valium" for its sedative properties.

- Safety: Generally safe; excessive use can lead to dizziness and withdrawal symptoms.

91. **Vitex (Chasteberry)**

- Origin: Mediterranean region and Central Asia.

- Uses: Hormonal balance, particularly in women.

- Benefits: Helps regulate menstrual cycles, and relieve symptoms of PMS and menopause.

- How to Use: Commonly taken as a supplement or extract.

- Interesting Fact: Historically used in monasteries to curb libido, hence the name 'Chasteberry'.

- Safety Information: This may interact with hormonal medications; not recommended during pregnancy.

92. White Willow Bark

- Origin: Europe and Asia.

- Uses: Natural pain relief and anti-inflammatory.

- Benefits: Contains salicin, which is similar to aspirin.

- How to Use: Available as a dried herb, tea, or supplement.

- Interesting Fact: Known as 'Nature's aspirin'.

- Safety Information: Should not be used by those allergic to aspirin or under 18 due to the risk of Reye's syndrome.

93. Wild Yam

- Origin: North America.

- Uses: Digestive health and menstrual cramp relief.

- Benefits: Contains diosgenin, used in estrogen therapy.

- How to Use: As a cream, supplement, or tea.

- Interesting Fact: Once used to make the first birth control pills.

- Safety Information: This can cause nausea; not recommended for pregnant or breastfeeding women.

94. Witch Hazel

- Origin: North America.

- Uses: Skin astringent and anti-inflammatory.

- Benefits: Helps with acne, skin irritation, and hemorrhoids.

- How to Use: Applied topically as a liquid extract, cream, or witch hazel water.

- Interesting Fact: Native Americans widely used it for medicinal purposes.

- Safety Information: Generally safe but may cause skin irritation in some people.

95. Yarrow

- Origin: Eurasia.

- Uses: Digestive aid and wound healing.

- Benefits: Helps stop bleeding and aids in digestion.

- How to Use: As a tea, tincture, or applied topically.

- Interesting Fact: Achilles supposedly used yarrow on his soldiers' wounds, hence its Latin name, Achillea.

- Safety Information: Can cause allergic reactions; not recommended during pregnancy.

96. Yellow Dock

- Origin: Europe and parts of Asia.

- Uses: Liver support and digestive aid.

- Benefits: Rich in iron, aids in detoxification.

- How to Use: Often taken as a supplement or used in salads.

- Interesting Fact: Historically used as a remedy for scurvy due to its high vitamin C content.

- Safety Information: Overuse can lead to mineral imbalance and constipation.

97. Yerba Mate

- Origin: South America.

- Uses: Energy boost and mental clarity.

- Benefits: Contains caffeine, and antioxidants.

- How to Use: Traditionally consumed as a brewed tea.

- Interesting Fact: Often shared socially in South America from a communal gourd.

- Safety Information: High consumption can lead to caffeine-related side effects.

98.**Yohimbe**

- Origin: Western and Central Africa.

- Uses: Circulatory health and energy boost.

- Benefits: Used for erectile dysfunction and weight loss.

- How to Use: As a supplement.

- Interesting Fact: The bark has been used traditionally as an aphrodisiac.

- Safety Information: Can cause serious side effects; consult a healthcare provider before use.

99.**Yucca**

- Origin: Americas and Caribbean.

- Uses: Anti-inflammatory and joint health.

- Benefits: Contains saponins, which may reduce arthritis symptoms.

- How to Use: As a supplement or in cooking.

- Interesting Fact: Yucca plants have been used by Native Americans for their fibers and medicinal properties.

- Safety Information: Excessive use can cause stomach upset.

100. **Zinc**

- Origin: Not applicable, as it is a mineral.

- Uses: Immune support and wound healing.

- Benefits: Essential for immune function and skin health.

- How to Use: Through diet or supplements.

- Interesting Fact: Zinc is the second-most abundant trace mineral in the human body after iron.

- Safety Information: Excessive intake can interfere with copper absorption and cause nausea.

101.   **Ziziphus (Jujube)**

- Origin: China.

- Uses: Sleep aid and stress relief.

- Benefits: Calming effect, sleep aids.

- How to Use: Eaten as a fruit, made into tea, or as a supplement.

- Interesting Fact: Jujube fruits are also known as red dates.

- Safety Information: Generally safe, but limited research on long-term use.

CHAPTER 4: ADVANCED HERBAL HEALING

Herbal healing, an ancient practice, has evolved significantly over the centuries. Originally based on trial and error, it has now embraced scientific methods to enhance its efficacy. Advanced herbal healing doesn't just involve the use of herbs; it's about understanding the intricate relationship between these natural remedies and human biology.

The Synergy of Herbs

At the core of advanced herbal healing is the understanding of herb synergy. Unlike conventional medicine, where a single active ingredient is often isolated, herbal medicine values the synergistic effect of various components within a plant. This synergy can enhance therapeutic benefits and reduce potential side effects. A classic example is the combination of echinacea and goldenseal, where echinacea boosts the immune system while goldenseal acts as a natural antibiotic.

Addressing Chronic Conditions

Herbal remedies can play a pivotal role in managing chronic conditions such as arthritis, diabetes, and heart disease. For instance, turmeric, with its active compound curcumin, is renowned for its anti-inflammatory properties, making it beneficial for arthritis patients. Similarly, herbs like Gymnema Sylvestre have shown promise in supporting blood sugar regulation in diabetic patients.

Advanced herbal healing is not a one-size-fits-all approach. It involves creating personalized herbal plans that consider an individual's unique health history, lifestyle, and current health status. A trained herbalist can help tailor a regimen that might include various herbs, dosages, and forms of administration, such as tinctures, capsules, or teas.

Diet and Lifestyle Integration

Advanced herbal healing also emphasizes the importance of diet and lifestyle. Herbs are most effective when complemented by a balanced diet, adequate hydration, regular physical activity, and stress management techniques. This integrated approach ensures that the body is in an optimal state to absorb and utilize the healing properties of herbs.

The Role of Adaptogens

Adaptogens are a unique class of herbs that help the body resist physical, chemical, and biological stressors. Herbs like Ashwagandha, Rhodiola, and Holy Basil are revered in advanced herbal healing for their ability to support adrenal health, improve stress response, and enhance overall vitality.

Future Trends and Research

The field of advanced herbal healing is continually evolving, with ongoing research uncovering new insights into plant-based therapies. There is a growing interest in the potential of herbs to support mental health, with studies exploring the effects of herbs like St. John's Wort and Lavender on conditions like depression and anxiety.

Safety and Efficacy

While herbal remedies are generally safe, they are potent and must be used responsibly. Understanding the proper dosages, potential side effects, and interactions with other medications is crucial. Consulting with healthcare professionals, especially for individuals with existing health conditions or those taking prescription medications, is always advised.

Sustainability and Ethical Sourcing

Advanced herbal healing also considers the sustainability and ethical sourcing of herbs. With the increasing demand for herbal products, it's essential to support practices that ensure the long-term viability of medicinal plants and respect the ecosystems from which they are harvested.

The Role of Traditional Knowledge

Respecting and integrating traditional herbal knowledge, especially from Indigenous and local communities, is a vital aspect of advanced herbal healing. Many modern herbal practices are rooted in centuries-old traditions, and acknowledging this lineage is crucial for an authentic and respectful approach to herbal medicine.

Finally, advanced herbal healing is about educating and empowering individuals to take charge of their health. By understanding how herbs work and how to use them effectively, individuals can make informed decisions about their health and well-being.

CHAPTER 5: BEYOND REMEDIES - A WHOLE LIFESTYLE

Creating a complete lifestyle that transcends mere remedies and encompasses a broader approach to well-being is essential for sustainable health and wellness. This comprehensive approach integrates herbal practices, exercise, mindfulness, and a personalized wellness plan. Here's an in-depth exploration:

Integrating Herbal Practices into Daily Life

Herbal remedies have been used for centuries, offering natural solutions to various health issues. Integrating these practices into daily life involves more than just consuming herbs; it's about embracing a philosophy that prioritizes natural, complete healing.

Understanding Herbs: To effectively incorporate herbs into your daily routine, it's crucial to understand their properties, benefits, and appropriate uses. Herbs like chamomile, lavender, and ginger are not just ingredients in remedies; they represent a connection to the earth and an understanding of its healing powers.

Kitchen as a Healing Space: Transform your kitchen into a healing space. Incorporate herbs into your cooking, not just for flavor, but for their health benefits. For instance, using turmeric in your dishes can provide anti-inflammatory benefits.

Creating Rituals: Establish rituals around herbal practices. This could be a morning tea ceremony with green tea for its antioxidant properties, or a nightly routine with a calming valerian root tincture.

The Role of Exercise in Holistic Healing

Physical activity is a cornerstone of complete health. It's not just about fitness; it's about creating harmony between the body and mind.

Exercise as Medicine: View exercise not as a chore, but as a form of medicine. Regular physical activity can reduce the risk of chronic diseases, improve mental health, and enhance the quality of life.

Mind-Body Connection: Choose exercises that strengthen the mind-body connection. Practices like yoga, tai chi, and Pilates are not just physical workouts; they also incorporate mindfulness, deep breathing, and meditation.

Nature and Exercise: Whenever possible, exercise outdoors. The connection with nature can amplify the benefits of physical activity, offering a sense of peace and grounding.

Mindfulness in Total Healing

Mindfulness is the practice of being present and fully engaged with whatever we're doing at the moment. In a complete lifestyle, mindfulness is a tool for healing and well-being.

Daily Mindfulness Practices: Incorporate mindfulness into everyday activities. This could be mindful eating, where you fully savor and appreciate your food, or mindful walking, where you pay attention to each step and your surroundings.

Stress Reduction: Mindfulness is a potent tool for stress reduction. Techniques like meditation, deep breathing exercises, and guided imagery can help calm the mind and reduce the physical symptoms of stress.

Emotional Balance: Mindfulness can foster emotional balance. By being present and aware, you're better equipped to handle emotional challenges and maintain a sense of inner peace.

Building a Personalized Herbal Wellness Plan

A personalized wellness plan is not a one-size-fits-all solution; it's a tailored approach to your unique health needs and goals.

Assessment: Start by assessing your health needs. Consider factors like your current health status, lifestyle, dietary habits, and any specific health goals or challenges.

Consultation with Professionals: While herbal remedies can be incredibly effective, it's important to consult with healthcare professionals, particularly if you have existing health conditions or are taking medication.

Customization: Customize your plan to include herbs that target your specific needs. For instance, if you struggle with sleep, herbs like valerian root or lavender might be beneficial.

Holistic Approach: Remember, a herbal wellness plan is just one component of a holistic lifestyle. It should be complemented with a balanced diet, regular exercise, and mindfulness practices.

Review and Adapt: Regularly review and adapt your plan. As your body and circumstances change, so too should your approach to wellness.

In conclusion, a holistic lifestyle that goes beyond remedies is about integrating natural health principles into every aspect of your life. It's a journey of understanding and connecting with your body, mind, and the natural world. By embracing herbal practices, exercise, mindfulness, and a personalized wellness plan, you create a sustainable path to health and well-being. Remember, the goal is not just to treat illness but to foster an environment where wellness thrives.

CONCLUSION: EMBRACING OVERALL HEALTH WITH INFORMED CAUTION

Resources and Further Reading

In the journey of exploring herbal remedies and overall health, continuous learning is key. While this book provides a substantial foundation, the field of natural medicine is vast and ever-evolving. Here are some resources for further reading and exploration:

1. **Books and Journals**: Beyond mainstream health literature, delve into specialized texts on herbal medicine. Look for authors with a blend of traditional knowledge and modern scientific research. Journals like the "Journal of Herbal Medicine" can offer peer-reviewed studies and recent discoveries.

2. **Online Resources**: Websites like the National Center for Complementary and Integrative Health (NCCIH) offer a wealth of information. Be cautious of sources, and prefer those that back their claims with research.

3. **Workshops and Seminars**: Hands-on workshops or seminars conducted by

experts can provide practical knowledge and a deeper understanding of herbology.

4. **Herbal Communities and Forums**: Engaging with a community of herbal enthusiasts can be enlightening. However, remember to cross-reference advice with reliable sources.

5. **Documentaries and Podcasts**: Visual and audio media can make learning more engaging. Look for documentaries and podcasts that approach herbal medicine both critically and respectfully.

6. **Traditional Knowledge Systems**: Explore texts and resources from traditional systems like Ayurveda, Traditional Chinese Medicine, or Native American Herbalism. Understanding different cultural approaches can provide a well-rounded perspective.

7. **Courses and Certifications**: If your interest is more than casual, consider formal education in herbal medicine. This can provide a structured and comprehensive understanding.

Safety Guidelines and Contraindications

While herbal remedies are natural, they are not without risks. Understanding safety guidelines and contraindications is crucial for responsible use.

1. **Consult Healthcare Providers**: Always consult with a healthcare professional before starting any new treatment, especially if you have existing health conditions or are on medication.

2. **Quality and Purity of Herbs**: Source herbs from reputable suppliers. Quality and purity are crucial for safety and efficacy.

3. **Dosage and Preparation**: Follow recommended dosages and preparation methods. Natural doesn't always mean safe in any amount or form.

4. **Understand Contraindications**: Some herbs may interact with medications or be unsuitable for certain conditions like pregnancy, breastfeeding, or chronic illnesses. Thorough research and professional advice are essential.

5. **Side Effects and Allergies**: Be aware of potential side effects and allergic reactions. Start with small doses to test for any adverse reactions.

6. **Sustainability**: Consider the ecological impact of using certain herbs. Opt for sustainably sourced herbs to protect biodiversity.

7. **Cultural Sensitivity**: Respect the cultural origins of herbal practices. Avoid appropriating or misrepresenting traditional knowledge.

8. **Keep Learning**: Stay updated on research and guidelines in herbal medicine. The field is dynamic, with new insights emerging regularly.

9. **Record Keeping**: Keep a journal of your herbal usage, including types, dosages, and any effects observed. This can be crucial for identifying what works best for you and for discussing your herbal practice with healthcare providers.

10. **Children and Elderly**: Exercise extra caution when considering herbal remedies for children or the elderly. Their bodies may react differently, and professional guidance is crucial.

11. **Emergency Situations**: Recognize when herbal remedies are not sufficient and

medical intervention is necessary. Herbal treatments are complementary and not a replacement for emergency medical care.

12. **Mind-Body Connection**: Remember that herbal remedies are part of a complete approach. Mental, emotional, and spiritual wellness are equally important.

In summary, the world of herbal remedies offers a fascinating blend of ancient wisdom and modern science. By responsibly sourcing and using herbs, consulting professionals, and continually educating oneself, it is possible to safely explore the myriad benefits these natural wonders offer. Remember, the journey towards health is not just about treating symptoms but embracing a holistic lifestyle that harmonizes the body, mind, and spirit.

Made in the USA
Monee, IL
30 January 2024

52669766R00066